LYME DISEASE RECOVERY MANUAL

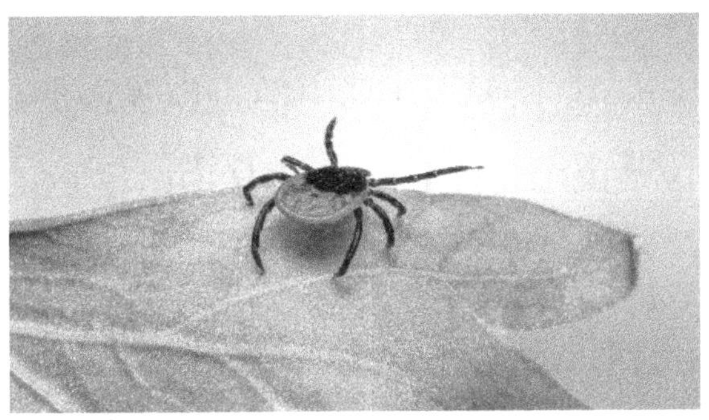

An Integrative Medical Guide to Daily Coping, Natural Remedies, and Nutritional Supports for People with Tick-Borne Illnesses

Thelma Pauley

Copyright © by Thelma Pauley 2024.

All rights reserved. Before this document is duplicated or reproduced in any manner, the publisher's consent must be gained. Therefore, the contents within can neither be stored electronically, transferred, nor kept in a database. Neither in Part nor full can the document be copied, scanned, faxed, or retained without approval from the publisher or creator.

TABLE OF CONTENT

CONCLUSION

Introduction

Welcome to the "Lyme Disease Recovery Manual," which is an all-in-one resource for getting your health and energy back after having Lyme disease. Most likely, you or someone you care about is dealing with the effects of Lyme disease since you are reading this book. You're not by yourself.

Lyme disease is a complicated illness that people don't always understand. It has the potential to impact every aspect of your life. can change every part of your life. The physical signs that make you tired and hurt, along with the mental toll of living with a long-term illness, can make the journey seem impossible to handle. But here's the good news: you have the power to take control of your health and thrive despite the obstacles.

In this manual, we'll start on a trip together—one of strength, education, and hope. We will give you the information and tools you need to handle the ups and downs of living with Lyme disease. We will also talk about a more complete way to heal that includes not only medical treatments but also changes to your lifestyle, natural cures, and nutritional support.

But before we dig into the strategies and solutions that will guide you toward healing, let's take a moment to understand what Lyme disease is and why this book was written. Lyme disease is caused by the bacterium Borrelia burgdorferi and is mainly spread through the bite of infected ticks. While early detection and treatment can lead to good outcomes, many people face difficulties in getting a correct diagnosis and effective care.

That's where this guidebook comes in. Drawing on the latest research, expert insights, and real-life experiences, we'll explain Lyme disease and provide you with practical help for controlling your symptoms, fighting for yourself in the healthcare system, and finding hope in the middle of hardship.

Whether you're newly identified, dealing with long-term symptoms, or helping a loved one on their journey, this manual is your path to resilience. Together, we'll manage the twists and turns of Lyme disease and emerge stronger, healthier, and more powerful than ever before.

So, let's start on this journey together. Are you ready to reclaim your health and find joy in daily life? Let's get started.

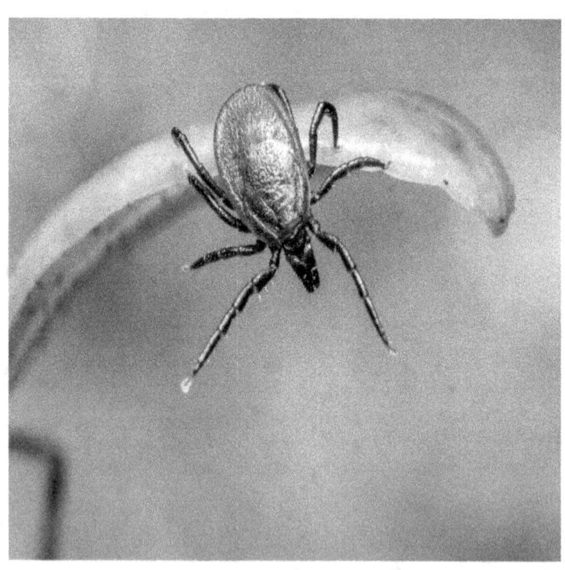

Chapter 1: Understanding Lyme Disease

Lyme disease is a sickness that you can get from a tick bite. It can make you feel very tired and give you a rash. Sometimes, it can even cause problems with your joints, heart, and brain. If you think you have Lyme disease, it's important to see a doctor who can give you medicine to help you feel better.

Causes and Transmission of Lyme Disease

Lyme disease is caused by the bacteria Borrelia burgdorferi. This bacteria is typically transmitted to humans by the bites of infected black-legged ticks, commonly known as deer ticks. Ticks become infected with the bacteria when they feed on diseased animals, such as mice or deer.

Lyme disease transmission is heavily reliant on the tick life cycle. Ticks progress through three phases of development: larvae, nymphs, and adults. To advance to the next level, they must first have a blood meal. When a tick is infected with Borrelia burgdorferi, the bacteria can be transmitted to a host during eating.

Ticks like woodland and grassy settings, where they may readily hook onto passing animals or people. When a tick attaches to a person and feeds on their blood, the bacteria can enter the circulation, potentially causing Lyme disease.

It's crucial to understand that not all ticks contain the bacteria that causes Lyme disease. Only a small minority of ticks carry Borrelia burgdorferi. However, the risk of developing Lyme disease varies with geographic location and the presence of infected ticks in the region.

Lyme disease is most commonly transmitted during the warm months when ticks are most active. However, infected ticks can be seen at any time of year, particularly in areas where the environment is generally mild throughout the year.

Lyme disease tends to spread more in places where there are lots of ticks and many of them carry the bacteria that cause the disease. These areas usually have more cases of Lyme disease reported every year. It's important to be extra cautious in these places and take steps to prevent tick bites.

Remember to wear long sleeves and pants when outdoors, use insect repellent, and check for ticks after spending time outside. By being aware of the risk factors and taking preventive measures, you can reduce the chances of getting Lyme disease and stay healthy.

Preventing tick bites is critical for minimizing the risk of Lyme disease transmission. Simple precautions, such as wearing long sleeves and trousers outside, applying DEET-containing insect repellents, and doing thorough tick inspections after spending time in tick-prone regions, can help avoid tick bites.

Tick removal should be done as soon as possible to avoid the spread of Lyme. Ticks normally need to be attached for at least 24 to 48 hours before transmitting the bacteria. As a result, eliminating ticks as soon as feasible can dramatically lower the risk of illness.

In conclusion, the bacteria Borrelia burgdorferi causes Lyme disease, which is typically transferred to people through the bite of infected black-legged ticks. Understanding the origins and transmission of Lyme disease is crucial for developing prevention strategies to lower the risk of infection.

Signs and Symptoms of Lyme Disease

Lyme disease can create a range of symptoms that might affect different sections of the body. It's vital to detect these indicators early to obtain the correct therapy and feel well.

One of the most common indicators of Lyme illness is a rash. This rash frequently looks like a bull's eye, with a red core surrounded by a clear region and then another red ring. Not everyone with Lyme disease gets this rash, but if you do, it's a strong warning that you need to visit a doctor.

Feeling fatigued and achy is another frequent symptom of Lyme disease. You can feel like you have the flu, with a fever, chills, headache, and muscular pains. These symptoms might come and go and could be modest at first but develop worse with time.

Lyme disease can also damage your joints, producing pain, swelling, and stiffness. Some persons with Lyme illness develop arthritis, especially in their knees. If you experience any joint discomfort or swelling that doesn't go away, it's crucial to notify your doctor.

In more severe cases, Lyme disease can impair your heart and nerve system. You can feel chest discomfort, abnormal heartbeats, or shortness of breath. Some patients also suffer numbness, tingling, or weakness in their arms and legs.

Other signs of Lyme disease might include:

Fatigue: Feeling weary all the time, even after having enough rest.

Poor Sleep: Trouble going to sleep staying asleep, or waking up feeling unrefreshed.

Cognitive Difficulties: Difficulty focusing, memory issues, or feeling foggy-headed.

Mood Changes: Feeling angry, worried, or sad.

If you experience any of these symptoms, especially after being outside in an area where ticks are widespread, it's crucial to consult a doctor straight once. Lyme disease may be treated with medications, especially if diagnosed early. But if left untreated, it might create more significant health concerns.

To prevent Lyme disease, it's crucial to make efforts to avoid tick bites. When you're outdoors, wear long sleeves and pants, apply insect repellent, and check your body for ticks after being outside. If you detect a tick stuck to your skin, remove it carefully with tweezers and disinfect the area with soap and water.

Lyme disease can produce a range of symptoms, including a rash, fever, weariness, joint pain, and more. If you develop any of these symptoms, especially after being bitten by a tick, visit a doctor straight away. With quick treatment, you can recover from Lyme disease and avert more catastrophic problems.

Diagnosing Lyme Disease

Diagnosing Lyme disease can be tricky since its symptoms can match those of other infections, and not everyone develops the telltale bull's-eye rash. However, there are various approaches that healthcare experts use to diagnose Lyme disease.

One of the key approaches to diagnosing Lyme disease is through a physical examination and medical history review. Your healthcare professional will inquire about your symptoms, any recent outside activities where you may have been exposed to ticks, and whether you've observed a rash. Be sure to report any recent tick bites or tick sightings, since this information can aid with diagnosis.

In addition to a physical exam, your healthcare practitioner may conduct laboratory testing to confirm the diagnosis of Lyme disease. The most often used test is the enzyme-linked immunosorbent assay (ELISA) test, which identifies antibodies generated by the body in response to the Lyme disease bacteria. If the ELISA test is positive or ambiguous, a confirmatory test called the Western blot test is frequently conducted.

It's crucial to note that laboratory testing for Lyme disease may not always be reliable, especially in the early stages of the infection. False-negative findings can arise if the tests are conducted too soon after the beginning of symptoms before the body has had a chance to build antibodies against the bacteria.

False-positive findings can sometimes occur, leading to undue stress and therapy.

In certain situations, healthcare personnel may diagnose Lyme disease based on clinical symptoms alone, especially if there is a documented history of tick contact and typical signs such as the bull's-eye rash. Treatment may be begun before laboratory test results are available to limit the spread of the illness and decrease the risk of consequences.

Overall, diagnosing Lyme disease needs a mix of clinical assessment, laboratory testing, and careful consideration of the patient's medical history and symptoms. If you believe you have Lyme disease or have been bitten by a tick, it's crucial to seek medical assistance quickly for examination and appropriate treatment.

Chapter 2: Daily Coping Strategies

Daily coping strategies are things you can do every day to help you deal with the challenges that come with Lyme disease. One key method is to listen to your body and rest when necessary. Moderate yourself and avoid trying to accomplish too much at once.

To avoid feeling overwhelmed, divide tasks down into smaller, more manageable steps. Surround yourself with helpful persons who understand your situation and can encourage you. Find activities that make you happy and feel good, such as spending time with loved ones, going for a stroll, or pursuing a passion.

Dealing with Fatigue and Pain

Living with Lyme disease can bring about challenges that affect your daily life, especially when it comes to dealing with fatigue and pain.

Fatigue, often described as extreme tiredness or lack of energy, can make even easy jobs feel overwhelming. Pain, whether it's joint pain, muscle aches, or headaches, can further add to the stress of handling Lyme disease symptoms. However, some methods and techniques can help you deal with fatigue and pain and improve your quality of life.

Understanding Fatigue

Fatigue is a common sign of Lyme disease and can vary in severity from person to person. It can feel like you're constantly drained of energy, making it difficult to focus, think, or participate in daily activities. Fatigue can be both physical and mental, affecting your body and your mind. It's important to spot the signs of fatigue and listen to your body when it's asking you to rest.

Coping with Fatigue

Managing fatigue takes a mix of self-care techniques and lifestyle changes. One of the most important things you can do is value rest. Allow yourself to take breaks throughout the day and listen to your body's cues when it needs to rest. Pace yourself and avoid overexertion by breaking jobs into smaller, more doable steps. Don't be afraid to ask for help from friends, family, or healthcare workers when you need it.

In addition to rest, adding light exercise into your schedule can help fight fatigue. Activities like walking, swimming, or yoga can help improve circulation, boost energy levels, and reduce feelings of tiredness. Start slowly and gradually increase the volume and length of your exercise as your energy levels allow.

Handling stress is also important for handling tiredness. Stress can worsen signs of fatigue and make it harder for your body to heal. Practice stress-reduction methods such as deep breathing, meditation, or awareness to help calm your mind and relax your body.

Understanding Pain

Pain is another common sign of Lyme disease and can appear in various ways, including joint pain, muscle aches, headaches, and nerve pain. Pain can range from mild to serious and can be constant or intermittent. It's important to pay attention to your body and share any pain signs with your healthcare provider.

Coping with Pain

Managing pain requires a diverse approach that tackles both physical and mental elements. Over-the-counter pain relievers such as acetaminophen or ibuprofen can help ease mild to severe pain. However, it's important to use these medications as advised and speak with your healthcare provider if you have any concerns.

In addition to medicine, alternative treatments such as acupuncture, massage, or physical therapy may provide relief from pain symptoms. These treatments can help improve circulation, reduce inflammation, and promote relaxation, which can help relieve pain.

Practicing good balance and body mechanics can also help lower pain sensations, especially if you experience joint or muscle pain. Avoiding repeated moves or activities that aggravate pain can help avoid further discomfort.

It's important to handle the emotional effect of pain as well. Chronic pain can take a toll on your mental health and well-being. Seek help from friends, family, or support groups who can offer understanding and guidance. Engage in activities that bring you joy and help remove you from pain, whether it's spending time with loved ones, chasing hobbies, or enjoying nature.

In conclusion, living with fatigue and pain is a major aspect of managing Lyme disease. By adding self-care techniques, living changes, and getting support from healthcare providers and loved ones, you can better deal with these symptoms and improve your overall quality of life.

Managing Mental Health

Managing mental health is a crucial part of dealing with Lyme illness. Dealing with a chronic condition, such as Lyme disease, may hurt your emotional health, causing feelings of worry, despair, or tension. However, some tactics and techniques can help you maintain and enhance your mental health as you deal with Lyme disease.

Understanding Mental Health Challenges

Living with Lyme disease can present a variety of mental health issues. The illness's unpredictability, impact on everyday life, and potential limits can all rise to emotions of frustration, melancholy, or solitude. Furthermore, physical symptoms of Lyme disease, such as weariness and discomfort, can worsen mental health problems and make it more difficult to deal with.

Coping Strategies For Mental Health

Managing mental health necessitates a proactive strategy that considers both the physical and emotional elements of Lyme disease. One of the most effective ways is to prioritize self-care. This involves obtaining adequate sleep, eating a healthy diet, and participating in regular physical activity. Taking care of your body might help you feel better and less anxious or depressed.

It is also vital to adopt stress management skills to assist cope with the problems of Lyme disease. Deep breathing techniques, mindfulness meditation, and yoga can all assist in relaxing your mind and body. Taking pauses and indulging in enjoyable activities can also assist in reducing stress and enhance your general well-being.

Seeking help from friends, family, or a mental health professional is also a vital part of managing mental health. Talking to someone who knows your situation might help you feel validated and supported. Furthermore, a mental health expert may provide coping skills and techniques to assist you in better managing your symptoms and improving your quality of life.

Participating in activities that offer relaxation and enjoyment can also benefit your mental health. Spending time outside, following hobbies, or engaging in creative activities might assist in diverting your attention away from negative thoughts and feelings. Finding purpose and meaning in your life, whether via volunteering, a job, or other activities, can improve your overall feeling of well-being.

Managing mental health is an essential part of dealing with Lyme illness. You may enhance your mental health and general quality of life by prioritizing self-care, using stress management skills, getting help from loved ones and specialists, and participating in pleasant activities. Remember, it's good to seek help when you need it, and you're not alone in your Lyme disease journey.

Maintaining Daily Activities

Maintaining regular activities while dealing with Lyme disease might be difficult, but it is vital to find methods to balance your duties and keep your independence. Despite the limitations provided by Lyme disease, you may continue to engage in meaningful activities and achieve your objectives by adopting tactics and modifications to your routine.

Understanding Lyme Disease's Impact on Daily Activities

Lyme disease can have a wide-ranging impact on daily living, including work, housework, social activities, and hobbies. Symptoms including exhaustion, discomfort, and cognitive challenges might make it difficult to complete things that were formerly simple or fun. However, with a few adaptations and concessions, you may continue to participate in activities that are meaningful to you.

Coping Strategies to Maintain Daily Activities

One approach for keeping up with everyday activities is to prioritize tasks and obligations depending on their significance and energy level. Identify the most important things that must be performed each day and devote your efforts accordingly. Pace yourself and take breaks as necessary to avoid weariness and save energy.

Breaking down projects into smaller, more manageable steps might help them feel less daunting and more realistic. Concentrate on doing one activity at a time rather than attempting to complete everything at once. This strategy might help you keep organized and feel accomplished during the day.

Using assistive equipment or adaptive strategies can also make daily tasks easier. For example, employing ergonomic equipment or assistive technologies can alleviate tension and make jobs simpler to complete. Modifying your surroundings, such as arranging furniture for better movement or using organizers to keep objects accessible, can also help with everyday tasks.

It's essential to discuss your wants and restrictions with others, whether they're family members, coworkers, or friends. Advocating for yourself and describing how Lyme illness impacts your capacity to engage in particular activities may help you get the support and understanding of others around you. Don't be hesitant to ask for help when you need it, and be willing to take it when it's granted.

Maintaining everyday activities while living with Lyme disease needs imagination, adaptability, and tenacity. Prioritizing things, breaking them down into manageable parts, using assistive technologies, and communicating your needs to others can allow you to continue engaging in meaningful activities while maintaining your freedom.

Remember to listen to your body, pace yourself, and acknowledge your victories, no matter how minor. With determination and adaptability, you may overcome the problems of Lyme disease and live a full life.

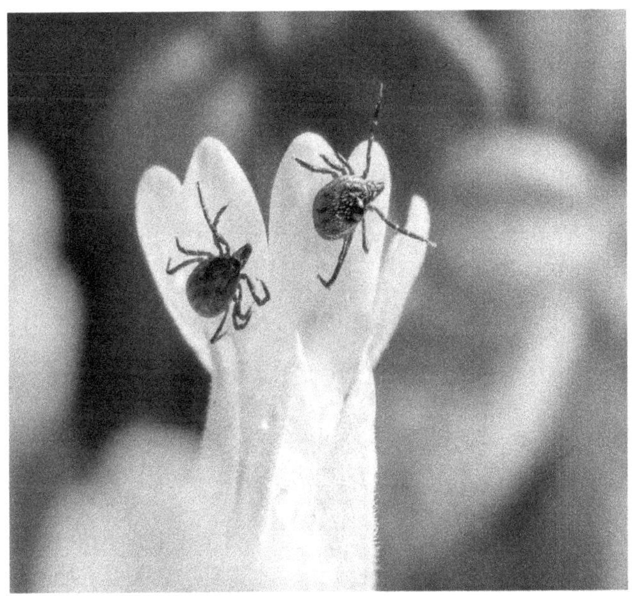

Chapter 3: Natural Remedies for Lyme Disease

Natural remedies for Lyme disease are treatments that use herbs, supplements, or lifestyle changes to help control symptoms and support the body's natural mending process. These solutions may include herbal supplements like garlic, turmeric, or cat's claw, which are thought to have anti-inflammatory and immune-boosting qualities.

Some people also find relief from symptoms by following a healthy diet, getting regular exercise, and lowering stress through methods like meditation or yoga. While natural cures can be helpful for some people, it's important to talk to a healthcare provider before trying any new treatment to ensure it's safe and effective for you.

Herbal Treatments for Lyme Disease

Herbal therapies are a popular way to manage Lyme disease symptoms and improve general health and well-being. Many herbs have been used for millennia in traditional medicine to stimulate the immune system, decrease inflammation, and combat infections. While herbal remedies are not a substitute for traditional medical care, they can be used as complementary therapies to help Lyme disease patients decrease symptoms and enhance their quality of life.

1. Garlic

Garlic is recognized for its strong antibacterial qualities, making it a popular choice for treating illnesses caused by bacteria such as Borrelia burgdorferi, the bacterium that causes Lyme disease. Garlic includes chemicals such as allicin, which have been demonstrated to suppress bacterial growth and improve immunological function. Including garlic in your diet or taking garlic supplements may strengthen your body's natural defenses against Lyme disease.

2. Cat's Claw

Uncaria tomentosa, or cat's claw, is a tropical vine that grows in the Amazon jungle. It has long been used in traditional medicine to treat a wide range of ailments, including infections and inflammation. Cat's claw includes chemicals known as oxindole alkaloids, which have been proven to have immune-stimulating and anti-inflammatory properties. According to certain research, a cat's claws may help decrease inflammation and improve symptoms in Lyme disease patients.

3. Japanese Knotweed

Japanese knotweed, also known as Polygonum cuspidatum or Hu Zhang in traditional Chinese medicine, is a perennial plant with potent anti-inflammatory and antibacterial effects. Japanese knotweed includes resveratrol, which has been found to limit Borrelia burgdorferi growth and decrease inflammation in the body. Some Lyme disease patients get relief from symptoms by including Japanese knotweed supplements in their treatment plan.

4. Andrographis

Andrographis, commonly known as Andrographis paniculata, is a bitter plant found in South Asian nations such as India and Sri Lanka. It has been used for ages in traditional Ayurvedic medicine to heal infections and boost immune function. Andrographis includes chemicals known as andrographolides, which have been shown to have antibacterial, anti-inflammatory, and immune-modulating properties. Some studies show that Andrographis may help minimize the intensity and duration of Lyme disease symptoms.

5. Samento

Samento, also known as Uncaria tomentosa or cat's claw, is a medicinal plant from the Amazon jungle. Indigenous people have used it for millennia to improve their immune systems and reduce inflammation. Samento includes chemicals known as pentacyclic oxindole alkaloids, which have been demonstrated to have antibacterial activity against Borrelia burgdorferi. Some Lyme disease patients report improved symptoms after using Samento supplements.

6. Astragalus

Astragalus is a traditional Chinese herb used for generations to boost immune function and increase general health and vigor. It includes substances known as polysaccharides, which have been demonstrated to activate the immune system and improve the body's capacity to fight infections. Astragalus may enhance the immune system and increase resistance to illnesses such as Lyme disease. Some Lyme disease patients include astragalus pills in their treatment program to boost immune function and general well-being.

7. Turmeric

Turmeric is a brilliant yellow spice made from the root of the Curcuma longa plant, which belongs to the ginger family. It includes curcumin, a substance with strong anti-inflammatory and antioxidant effects. Turmeric has been used for millennia in traditional Ayurvedic and Chinese medicine to treat a wide range of ailments, including infections and inflammation. Some Lyme disease patients experience relief from symptoms by taking turmeric pills or including turmeric in their diet.

Herbal remedies provide a natural and holistic approach to controlling Lyme disease symptoms while also promoting general health and well-being.

While herbal therapies might be effective for some people, it's critical to talk with a doctor before beginning any new treatment plan, especially if you're already on prescription or have underlying health issues. Working with a trained practitioner and combining herbal remedies into a complete treatment plan can help you manage Lyme disease symptoms and improve your quality of life.

Homeopathic Remedies for Lyme Disease

Homeopathy is a holistic method of medicine that uses natural substances to promote the body's internal healing ability. Homeopathic remedies are prepared from highly diluted substances derived from plants, minerals, or animals and are prescribed based on the principle of "like cures like," meaning that a substance that causes symptoms in a healthy person can be used to treat similar symptoms in a person with an illness.

While homeopathy is controversial and its success is discussed, some people with Lyme disease find relief from symptoms and improvement in their general well-being through homeopathic treatment. In this guide, we will explore different homeopathic medicines widely used for Lyme disease and their possible benefits.

1. Marsh Tea (Ledum palustre)

Ledum palustre, also known as marsh tea or wild

rosemary, is a homeopathic remedy widely used for Lyme disease, especially in the early stages. It is produced from the flowering plant Ledum palustre, which is native to cold, swampy areas of North America, Europe, and Asia.

Ledum is recommended for people who experience puncture wounds or bug bites, such as those caused by ticks, and who show symptoms such as redness, swelling, and stiffness in the affected area. It is also used to help avoid the growth of Lyme disease symptoms after a tick bite.

2. Honeybee (Apis mellifica)

Apis mellifica, or honeybee, is a homeopathic medicine made from the venom of the honeybee. It is recommended for people with Lyme disease who experience symptoms such as swelling, redness, and burning or stinging pain, similar to a bee sting. Apis is often used to help reduce signs of inflammation and swelling associated with Lyme disease, especially in the joints or skin. It may also be helpful for people who experience allergic responses to bee stings or bug bites.

3. Arsenic (Arsenicum album)

Arsenicum album, or arsenic, is a homeopathic remedy widely used for a range of health problems, including Lyme disease. It is suggested for people who experience symptoms such as weakness, fatigue, anxiety, restlessness, and digestive problems.

Arsenicum is often used to help reduce signs of exhaustion and malaise linked with Lyme disease, as well as to support the body's natural detoxification processes. It may also be helpful for people who experience gastrointestinal complaints such as nausea, vomiting, diarrhea, or abdominal pain.

4. Poison Ivy (Rhus Toxicodendron)

Rhus Toxicodendron, or poison ivy, is a homeopathic remedy made from the toxic plant poison ivy. It is recommended for people with Lyme disease who experience symptoms such as stiffness, soreness, and restlessness, especially in the muscles and joints.

Rhus tox is often used to help reduce symptoms of arthritis, myalgia, and rheumatic pain linked with Lyme disease. It may also be helpful for people who experience symptoms such as itching, burning, or blistering of the skin, similar to poison ivy disease.

5. Deadly Nightshade (Belladonna)

Belladonna, or dangerous nightshade, is a homeopathic medicine drawn from the toxic plant belladonna. It is recommended for people with Lyme disease who experience symptoms such as rapid start of fever, strong heat, redness, and throbbing pain, similar to a sunburn. Belladonna is often used to help alleviate signs of acute inflammation and fever linked with Lyme disease, as well as to support the body's natural healing reaction. It may also be helpful for people who experience symptoms such as headache, confusion, or sensitivity to light and noise.

6. Borrelia burgdorferi Nosode

Borrelia burgdorferi nosode is a homeopathic remedy made from a dilution of the bacteria Borrelia burgdorferi, which causes Lyme disease. It is used to help stimulate the body's immune reaction and promote healing in people with Lyme disease. Borrelia nosode is recommended for people who have been identified with Lyme disease or who have a history of exposure to ticks carrying the Lyme disease bacteria. It may help alleviate symptoms linked with Lyme disease and support the body's natural ability to fight off the illness.

Homeopathic remedies offer a natural and holistic method of handling Lyme disease symptoms and supporting general health and well-being. While homeopathy is controversial and its usefulness is debated, some people with Lyme disease find relief from symptoms and change in their quality of life through homeopathic treatment.

It's important to work with a trained homeopathic practitioner who can tailor treatment to your individual needs and watch your progress over time. By incorporating homeopathic remedies as part of a complete treatment plan, you can better handle Lyme disease symptoms and improve your general well-being.

Essential Oils For Lyme Disease

Essential oils are concentrated plant extracts that include the aromatic ingredients and medicinal capabilities of the plants from which they originate. While essential oils cannot replace conventional medical treatment, they can be utilized as complementary therapies to help control symptoms and promote general well-being in people with Lyme disease. In this article, we'll look at the numerous essential oils that are widely used to treat Lyme disease and their possible advantages.

1. Lavender Oil

Lavender oil is well-known for its calming and soothing characteristics, making it a popular option for treating Lyme disease-related stress, anxiety, and sleeplessness. It possesses anti-inflammatory and analgesic qualities, which may aid in relieving muscular and joint discomfort. Lavender oil can be used directly on the skin, mixed with a carrier oil, or diffused in the air to promote relaxation and enhance sleep.

2. Peppermint Oil

Peppermint oil is stimulating and refreshing, with cooling characteristics that might help reduce Lyme disease-related headaches, muscular strain, and exhaustion. It possesses analgesic and anti-inflammatory properties, which may help alleviate pain and suffering. Peppermint oil can be used directly on one temple, neck, or other painful regions, mixed with a crier oil, or breathed through steam inhalation or a diffuser to improve alertness and mental clarity.

3. Frankincense Oil

Frankincense oil is valued for its anti-inflammatory and immune-boosting characteristics, making it an effective tool for controlling Lyme disease symptoms. It has been used in traditional medicine for generations to aid healing and decrease inflammation. Frankincense oil can be used directly to inflamed regions, mixed with carrier oil, or diffused into the air to promote general health and boost the body's natural healing processes.

4. Tea Tree Oil

Tea tree oil is well-known for its antibacterial and antiseptic characteristics, which make it a useful treatment for Lyme disease-related skin infections, rashes, and sores. It has been demonstrated to suppress the growth of bacteria, fungi, and viruses, making it an important component in natural first aid kits. Tea tree oil can be used directly on the skin, diluted with a carrier oil, or mixed into bath water to cleanse and soothe sore skin.

5. Eucalyptus Oil

Eucalyptus oil is well-known for its respiratory benefits and potential to alleviate Lyme disease-related congestion, coughing, and sinusitis symptoms. It possesses expectorant and decongestant effects, which can help clear the airways and make breathing easier. Eucalyptus oil can be breathed as steam, mixed with a carrier oil, and applied topically to the chest or throat, or diffused into the air to relieve respiratory symptoms and enhance overall respiratory health.

6. Rosemary Oil

Rosemary oil is energetic and stimulating, and it has cognitive-enhancing characteristics that can help you focus, concentrate, and think more clearly. It possesses antioxidant and anti-inflammatory properties, which may help lessen the inflammation and suffering associated with Lyme disease. Rosemary oil can be diffused in the air, mixed with a crier oil and applied topically to the temples or wrists, or breathed via steam inhalation to improve mental alertness and cognitive performance.

7. Oregano Oil

Oregano oil is well-known for its significant antibacterial qualities, which make it useful against bacterial illnesses such as Borrelia burgdorferi, the bacterium that causes Lyme disease. It also possesses anti-inflammatory and immune-boosting effects, which can help decrease inflammation and strengthen the body's natural defenses.

8. Thyme Oil

Thyme oil is another powerful antibacterial agent that can help treat Lyme disease-related bacterial infections. It includes chemicals such as thymol and carvacrol, which have been demonstrated to suppress bacterial development while promoting healing. Thyme oil contains analgesic qualities that can help relieve pain and suffering.

9. Clove Oil

Clove oil is high in antioxidants and has significant

antibacterial qualities, making it beneficial against both bacterial and fungal illnesses. It also contains analgesic effects that can help alleviate the pain and inflammation caused by Lyme disease. Clove oil can be very effective in alleviating joint pain and stiffness.

In addition to the widely used essential oils mentioned earlier, several other essential oils may offer benefits for people managing Lyme disease symptoms. These essential oils, known for their therapeutic qualities, can support standard treatment methods and provide relief from various symptoms such as pain, inflammation, and mental discomfort.

Let's study these extra essential oils and their possible additions to Lyme disease management.

1. Lemongrass Oil

Lemongrass oil is produced from the Lemongrass plant and is famous for its antimicrobial and immune-supportive qualities. Rich in compounds like citral and geraniol, Lemongrass oil has been studied for its usefulness against different bacteria and fungi, making it possibly useful in combating infections linked with Lyme disease. Its uplifting citrusy flavor can also provide a refreshing boost, boosting mental focus and energy.

2. Geranium Oil

Geranium oil, taken from the leaves and flowers of the Geranium plant, offers a range of therapeutic effects. With its anti-inflammatory and analgesic effects, Geranium oil may help alleviate pain and reduce inflammation in people with Lyme disease. Additionally, its balancing effect on emotions can provide mental support, easing feelings of stress and worry widely experienced by those managing chronic health conditions.

3. Helichrysum Oil

Helichrysum oil is prized for its potent anti-inflammatory and wound-healing qualities, making it a valuable addition to the toolkit for people with Lyme disease. Rich in compounds like curcumin and alpha-pinene, Helichrysum oil can help lower inflammation, promote tissue repair, and support general skin health. Its sweet, earthy scent may also offer relaxation and mental comfort.

4. Cypress Oil

Cypress oil, taken from the branches of the Cypress tree, contains astringent and vasoconstrictive qualities, making it helpful for improving circulation and reducing swelling. Individuals with Lyme disease who experience joint pain and inflammation may find relief from Cypress oil's ability to relieve discomfort and promote movement. Its fresh, woody smell can also give a feeling of security and grounding.

5. Myrrh Oil

Myrrh oil, produced from the resin of the Myrrh tree, boasts powerful anti-inflammatory and antimicrobial properties, making it an excellent choice for people seeking natural remedies for Lyme disease control. With its ability to reduce inflammation and fight infections, Myrrh oil can support the body's healing process and promote general wellness. Its warm, resinous flavor can evoke feelings of comfort and peace.

6. Juniper Berry Oil

Juniper berry oil is known for its detoxifying and diuretic effects, making it helpful for supporting the body's natural detoxification processes and promoting kidney function. With its ability to promote urine output and remove toxins, Juniper berry oil can aid in flushing out harmful substances from the body, possibly improving general health and well-being. Its fresh, woody fragrance can also uplift the mood and promote mental focus.

7. Bergamot Oil

Bergamot oil, extracted from the peel of the Bergamot fruit, offers a refreshing citrus aroma and a range of medicinal effects. With its uplifting and mood-enhancing effects, Bergamot oil can help alleviate feelings of stress, worry, and sadness often linked with chronic health conditions like Lyme disease. Its bright, citrusy scent can boost the mood and support mental balance.

8. Ginger Oil

Ginger oil, produced from the rhizome of the Ginger plant, possesses analgesic and anti-inflammatory qualities, making it useful for managing pain and inflammation in people with Lyme disease. Whether applied topically or inhaled aromatically, Ginger oil can help relieve pain and promote relaxation. Its warm, spicy scent can also excite the senses and improve general well-being.

While these additional essential oils offer potential therapeutic benefits for individuals with Lyme disease, it's important to use them safely and speak with a qualified healthcare provider or aromatherapist before adding them to your treatment routine.

Essential oils should be properly diluted and used with care, especially for people with sensitive skin or underlying health problems. With careful thought and direction, essential oils can be useful allies in managing Lyme disease symptoms and promoting general health and well-being.

Essential oils provide a natural and holistic way to control Lyme disease symptoms while also promoting general health and well-being. While essential oils can be useful to some people, it's crucial to use them responsibly and check with a certified healthcare practitioner before beginning any new treatment program, especially if you have underlying health concerns, are pregnant, or are nursing Essential oils, when combined with a thorough treatment plan, can help you manage Lyme disease symptoms and improve your overall quality of life.

Chapter 4: Nutritional Support

Nutritional support plays a crucial role in managing Lyme disease, as a well-balanced diet can help strengthen the immune system, reduce inflammation, and support overall health. Including nutrient-rich foods such as fruits, vegetables, lean proteins, and healthy fats can provide essential vitamins, minerals, and antioxidants to promote healing and reduce symptoms.

Additionally, certain supplements like omega-3 fatty acids, probiotics, and vitamin D may offer further support in managing Lyme disease symptoms and enhancing overall well-being. Working with a healthcare provider or nutritionist to develop a personalized nutrition plan can optimize treatment outcomes and improve quality of life.

Importance of Diet in Lyme Disease

Lyme disease, caused by the bacteria Borrelia burgdorferi and transmitted by the bite of infected black-legged ticks, can produce a variety of symptoms affecting several organ systems. While antibiotic medication is the primary treatment for Lyme disease, eating a healthy diet can help manage symptoms, boost the immune system, and promote overall well-being.

1. Anti-inflammatory Foods

Inflammation is a defining characteristic of Lyme disease, leading to symptoms including joint discomfort, exhaustion, and cognitive impairment. Consuming an anti-inflammatory diet high in fruits, vegetables, whole grains, healthy fats, and lean meats will help reduce inflammation and symptoms.

Omega-3 fatty acid-rich foods include fatty fish (salmon, mackerel, sardines), flaxseeds, chia seeds, and walnuts, which have significant anti-inflammatory qualities and may help decrease joint discomfort and swelling. Incorporating a variety of colorful fruits and vegetables, such as berries, leafy greens, tomatoes, and bell peppers, delivers antioxidants that fight inflammation and promote cell health.

2. Gut Health

The gut microbiota influences immune function and general health. Lyme disease and antibiotic therapy can upset the balance of gut flora, resulting in gastrointestinal symptoms such as bloating, gas, and diarrhea. Consuming probiotic-rich foods like yogurt, kefir, sauerkraut, kimchi, and kombucha can help replenish gut flora and improve digestive health. Furthermore, prebiotic foods such as garlic, onions, leeks, asparagus, and bananas support beneficial gut bacteria, promoting microbiome diversity and resilience.

3. Immune-boosting nutrients

Individuals with Lyme disease must support their

immune systems since a strong immune response is vital for treating the illness and avoiding consequences. Vitamin C, vitamin D, zinc, and selenium are all essential nutrients for immunological function and may be received through a well-balanced diet.

Citrus fruits, strawberries, kiwi, bell peppers, and broccoli are high in vitamin C, which improves immune cell activity and promotes wound healing. Vitamin D, which is present in fatty fish, fortified dairy products, eggs, and sunshine, regulates immune responses and may lessen the incidence of autoimmune reactions in Lyme disease.

Zinc, which is rich in shellfish, red meat, chicken, beans, nuts, and seeds, promotes immune cell formation and function, whereas selenium, found in Brazil nuts, seafood, and whole grains, boosts antioxidant defenses and immunological regulation.

4. Protein-Rich Foods

Protein is required for tissue repair, muscle

maintenance, and immunological function, making it an important part of the Lyme disease diet. Incorporating lean protein sources like poultry, fish, lean cattle, eggs, tofu, tempeh, and legumes into meals and snacks can aid with recovery and general well-being. Protein also helps to balance blood sugar levels and increase satiety, lowering the likelihood of energy crashes and providing sustainable energy throughout the day.

5. Hydration

Proper hydration is essential for Lyme disease patients since dehydration can increase symptoms including tiredness, headaches, and cognitive problems. Drinking enough water throughout the day helps you stay hydrated, aids detoxification processes, and improves nutrient absorption. Aim to drink at least eight glasses of water every day, and adapt accordingly based on activity level, environment, and personal needs. Herbal teas, coconut water, and electrolyte-rich drinks can also help with hydration and offer extra health advantages.

6. Avoiding Trigger Foods

Some Lyme disease patients may have food sensitivities or intolerances, which can worsen symptoms and slow healing. Common trigger foods include gluten-containing grains (wheat, barley, and rye), dairy products, processed meals, sugar, caffeine, alcohol, and artificial additives.

Keeping a food diary and noting how different meals impact symptoms might help you discover trigger foods and make better nutritional choices. Eliminating or limiting trigger foods and substituting full, unprocessed meals can help reduce symptom flare-ups and improve overall health.

Finally, adopting a nutritious diet adapted to individual needs can be an effective part of Lyme disease care. Individuals with Lyme disease may improve their nutritional status, reduce symptoms, and promote overall well-being by concentrating on anti-inflammatory meals, supporting gut health, ingesting immune-boosting nutrients, including protein-rich foods, staying hydrated, and avoiding trigger foods.

It is crucial to collaborate with a healthcare physician or registered dietitian to create a tailored nutrition plan that meets unique symptoms, dietary preferences, and health objectives. Individuals with Lyme disease can improve their quality of life and help their recovery by eating a well-balanced diet and adopting a holistic approach to well-being.

Nutritious Foods for Lyme Disease Management

When coping with Lyme disease, a well-balanced diet can help promote the body's healing process, strengthen the immune system, and reduce symptoms. By including a range of nutrient-dense foods in your daily diet, you may provide your body with the vitamins, minerals, antioxidants, and other substances it requires to flourish. To properly treat Lyme disease, consider include the following items in your diet:

1. Lean Protein Sources

Consuming lean protein sources is essential for muscle regeneration, immunological function, and general health. Choose lean meats like chicken, turkey, and lean cuts of beef or pork. Fish, especially fatty fish such as salmon, mackerel, and trout, contain omega-3 fatty acids, which have anti-inflammatory qualities. Plant-based protein foods such as beans, lentils, tofu, and edamame are also great choices for vegetarians and vegans.

2. Colorful Fruits and Vegetables

Fruits and vegetables provide vital vitamins, minerals, antioxidants, and phytonutrients that can help reduce inflammation, enhance immunity, and promote healing. Try to eat a range of bright fruits and vegetables, such as berries, citrus fruits, leafy greens, bell peppers, tomatoes, carrots, and sweet potatoes. These foods have a diverse set of nutrients that promote general health and well-being.

3. Whole Grains

Whole grains provide fiber, vitamins, minerals, and antioxidants that promote digestive health, control blood sugar levels, and reduce inflammation. Select whole grains such as brown rice, quinoa, barley, oats, whole wheat, and buckwheat. These grains are high in fiber and other nutrients that help you feel full and maintain good health over time.

4. Healthy Fats

Healthy fats are essential for maintaining brain function, decreasing inflammation, and improving general well-being. Avocados, almonds, seeds, olive oil, and fatty fish such as salmon and mackerel are also good sources of healthful fat. These foods include omega-3 fatty acids, which are anti-inflammatory and may help lessen Lyme disease symptoms.

5. Foods with High Probiotic Content

Supporting gut health is important for Lyme disease patients since the gut plays an important role in immune function and general health. Consuming probiotic-rich foods can help maintain a healthy balance of gut flora and improve digestive health. Incorporate foods rich in probiotics like yogurt, kefir, sauerkraut, kimchi, and kombucha into your diet.

6. Herbs & Spices

Herbs and spices not only enhance the flavor of your food, but they also give several health advantages. Many herbs and spices have anti-inflammatory, antioxidant, and immune-boosting compounds that can benefit general health and well-being. To add taste and nutritional value to your meals, use herbs and spices such as turmeric, ginger, garlic, cinnamon, and oregano.

7. Hydration

Staying hydrated is critical for general health and

well-being, particularly for people with Lyme disease. Adequate hydration promotes detoxification, digestion, nutritional absorption, and general cell function. To maintain appropriate hydration levels, drink lots of water throughout the day and incorporate hydrating items such as fruits, vegetables, and herbal teas into your diet.

8. Antioxidant-Rich Foods

Consuming antioxidant-rich foods can help counteract oxidative stress, decrease inflammation, and promote general health. Include antioxidant-rich foods such as berries, cherries, grapes, spinach, kale, broccoli, and dark chocolate.

By including these nutrient-dense foods in your diet, you may provide your body with the nutrition it requires to improve immunological function, reduce inflammation, and promote healing. Furthermore, eating a diverse and balanced diet can help boost energy levels, improve general well-being, and aid in long-term health and recovery.

Foods to Avoid for Lyme Disease Management

When managing Lyme disease, it's required to consider not just the foods you eat, but also the ones you should avoid. Certain foods might worsen symptoms, cause inflammation, or impair immunological function, reducing your body's capacity to heal and recover. By reducing or eliminating these harmful items from your diet, you can improve your health and well-being.

Here are some items to avoid while managing Lyme disease:

1. Processed Foods

Processed meals are frequently heavy in harmful fats, carbohydrates, salt, and artificial additives, which can promote inflammation, disturb gastrointestinal health, and weaken the immune system. Avoid packaged snacks, sugary cereals, fast meals, fried foods, and processed meats, since these might aggravate symptoms and slow healing.

2. Sugar and Refined Carbohydrates

Highly processed sugars and refined carbs can cause blood sugar increases, increase inflammation, and impair the immune system. Candy, soda, pastries, white bread, white rice, and sugary desserts should be avoided since they can increase Lyme disease symptoms such as weariness, joint discomfort, and brain fog.

3. Gluten-containing Grains

Gluten, a protein present in wheat, barley, rye, and other grains, can cause inflammation and worsen digestive problems in certain people, including those with Lyme disease. Avoid gluten-containing grains, such as wheat-based bread, pasta, cereal, and baked goods, and instead choose gluten-free options like quinoa, brown rice, and gluten-free oats.

4. Dairy Products

Dairy items such as milk, cheese, and yogurt may be harmful to certain Lyme disease patients because they can cause inflammation, digestive problems, and immune system malfunction. Furthermore, dairy products might be difficult to digest for people who have poor gut health. Consider limiting or eliminating dairy from your diet in favor of dairy-free options such as almond milk, coconut yogurt, and cheese.

5. Alcohol

Alcohol can decrease immunological function, disturb sleep patterns, and aggravate Lyme disease symptoms including weariness and cognitive fog. Furthermore, drinking can impair drug efficiency and liver function, reducing the body's capacity to cleanse and recover. Limit or avoid alcohol use when treating Lyme disease to improve general health and well-being.

6. Caffeine

Caffeinated beverages such as coffee, tea, and energy drinks can aggravate Lyme disease symptoms including sleeplessness, anxiety, and heart palpitations. Caffeine can also alter adrenal function, aggravate exhaustion, and cause hormonal imbalances. Consider lowering or eliminating caffeine from your diet in favor of caffeine-free options such as herbal tea or decaf coffee.

7. Artificial Additives

Artificial sweeteners, preservatives, and food colorings may cause inflammation, upset gut health, and worsen Lyme disease symptoms. Avoid meals and drinks that contain artificial additives, and if feasible, choose whole, minimally processed foods.

8. Fish with High Mercury Levels

Certain species of fish, particularly large predatory fish such as sharks, swordfish, king mackerel, and tilefish, may contain high amounts of mercury, which can be damaging to health, particularly for

Lyme disease patients. Mercury can damage immunological function and brain health, worsening symptoms including weariness, cognitive impairment, and joint pain. To avoid mercury exposure, choose low-mercury seafood such as salmon, sardines, trout, and anchovies.

9. Food Allergens

Some people with Lyme disease may have food allergies or sensitivities, which aggravate symptoms and slow healing. Common food allergies include nuts, shellfish, soy, eggs, and some fruits and vegetables. Pay attention to how various foods impact your symptoms, and try removing probable allergens from your diet to help you identify triggers and manage symptoms.

In addition to the above-indicated foods, there are numerous more products that patients with Lyme disease may benefit from avoiding to manage symptoms efficiently and maintain overall health. Here are some other things to consider removing or limiting in your diet:

1. Nightshade Vegetables

Nightshade vegetables including tomatoes, peppers, eggplants, and potatoes contain alkaloids that may aggravate inflammation and contribute to joint discomfort in certain patients with Lyme disease. While not everyone will respond poorly to nightshades, some may find symptom alleviation by limiting their consumption or removing them from their diet temporarily.

2. High-Sugar Fruits

While fruits are usually considered healthful, certain types are heavier in sugar than others and may contribute to surges in blood sugar levels and worsen symptoms like exhaustion and brain fog. Examples of high-sugar fruits include bananas, grapes, mangoes, and pineapples. Opt for lower-sugar choices like berries, apples, and citrus fruits to help stabilize blood sugar levels and limit symptom flare-ups.

3. High-Salt Foods

Foods rich in salt can contribute to water retention, bloating, and raised blood pressure, which may worsen symptoms like joint pain and exhaustion in those with Lyme disease. Avoid processed and packaged meals like canned soups, salty snacks, and deli meats, which are generally high in sodium. Instead, flavor your meals with herbs, spices, and natural seasonings to minimize salt intake and enhance overall health.

4. Artificial Sweeteners

Artificial sweeteners including aspartame, sucralose, and saccharin are often found in diet drinks, sugar-free goods, and processed meals marketed as "low-calorie" or "sugar-free." These artificial sweeteners may disturb gut health, induce inflammation, and contribute to digestive disorders in certain persons. Opt for natural sweeteners like stevia, honey, or maple syrup in moderation, or pick meals and beverages that are free from artificial sweeteners.

5. Processed Meats

Processed meats like bacon, sausage, hot dogs, and deli meats generally include chemicals, preservatives, and high levels of salt, which can lead to inflammation and weaken immune function. Additionally, these meats may include nitrates and nitrites, which have been linked to an elevated risk of certain health issues. Choose lean, unprocessed sources of protein like fowl, fish, tofu, or lentils instead.

6. Highly Acidic Foods

Highly acidic meals like citrus fruits, vinegar, and acidic beverages like coffee and alcohol may increase symptoms like acid reflux, heartburn, and digestive pain in certain persons with Lyme disease. While these foods can be enjoyed in moderation by some people, others may find comfort in lowering their consumption or eliminating them, especially during periods of symptom flare-ups.

7. Allergenic Foods

Food allergies or sensitivities can activate immunological responses and increase symptoms in persons with Lyme disease. Common allergic foods include gluten, dairy, soy, eggs, nuts, and shellfish. Consider removing probable allergens from your diet temporarily and returning them one at a time to discover triggers and help symptom management.

Individuals with Lyme disease can improve their health by avoiding these harmful foods and eating a healthy diet. Listen to your body, observe how different foods influence your symptoms, and collaborate with a healthcare physician or registered dietitian to create a tailored nutrition plan that suits your specific needs while promoting healing and recovery.

Chapter 5: Seeking Medical Treatment

Seeking medical care is vital for patients with Lyme disease to successfully manage symptoms, minimize complications, and improve recovery. Consultation with a healthcare professional, ideally knowledgeable in treating tick-borne infections, can lead to early diagnosis and proper treatment. Medical interventions may include medicines to remove the bacterial infection, pain management methods to ease discomfort, and supportive therapy to address symptoms such as exhaustion and cognitive impairment. Regular follow-up consultations and open contact with healthcare professionals provide continuing monitoring of progress and adjustment of treatment regimens as needed, eventually ensuring optimal health outcomes for patients with Lyme disease.

Conventional Treatment Options for Lyme Disease

Lyme disease, caused by the bacteria Borrelia burgdorferi and transmitted by the bite of infected black-legged ticks, can produce a variety of symptoms affecting several organ systems. While early identification and treatment are critical for avoiding problems, people with Lyme disease may benefit from several traditional treatments targeted at eliminating the infection, treating symptoms, and improving recovery.

Here are some of the major conventional treatment options for Lyme disease.

1. Antibiotics

Antibiotics are the primary treatment for Lyme disease, especially in the early stages of illness. The kind, dose, and length of antibiotics recommended may differ based on the illness stage, severity of symptoms, and specific patient characteristics. Doxycycline, amoxicillin, and cefuroxime axetil are common antibiotics recommended to treat Lyme disease. These medicines operate by eliminating the Borrelia burgdorferi germ from the body and preventing the infection from progressing.

2. Duration of Antibiotic Treatment

The length of antibiotic therapy for Lyme disease varies based on various factors, including illness stage, symptom intensity, and individual patient characteristics. A course of oral antibiotics for early-stage Lyme disease lasts around two to four weeks. In situations of disseminated or late-stage Lyme disease, intravenous (IV) antibiotics may be required for a longer period, ranging from a few weeks to months. To guarantee infection eradication and avoid recurrence, finish the whole course of antibiotics as advised by a healthcare practitioner.

3. Symptom Management

In addition to antibiotic medication, people with Lyme disease may need symptomatic treatment to relieve pain and enhance their quality of life.

Depending on the symptoms, healthcare practitioners may give nonsteroidal anti-inflammatory medicines (NSAIDs) for pain and inflammation, antihistamines for allergic responses, or corticosteroids for severe inflammation or neurological issues. Lifestyle changes, dietary alterations, physical therapy, and complementary therapies such as acupuncture or massage therapy are all possible symptom management techniques.

4. Supportive Therapy

Supportive therapy can help manage Lyme disease symptoms and improve general well-being. These therapies may include intravenous (IV) fluids to stay hydrated, nutritional assistance to guarantee proper nutrient intake, and restorative therapies to alleviate weariness and improve recovery. Physical, occupational, and speech therapy may be suggested to treat particular symptoms such as joint pain, muscular weakness, and cognitive impairment. Mental health support services, such as counseling or psychotherapy, can also help people deal with the emotional and psychological effects of Lyme disease.

5. Follow-Up Care

Individuals receiving Lyme disease therapy must attend regular follow-up sessions with their healthcare specialists. These sessions let healthcare practitioners track progress, evaluate treatment outcomes, and make any required changes to the treatment plan. Physical examinations, laboratory tests, imaging investigations, and talks about current symptoms and treatment choices may all be part of the follow-up care. Open communication between patients and healthcare professionals is critical for achieving the best treatment outcomes and resolving any issues or questions that may emerge throughout therapy.

6. Prevention Strategies

Prevention is essential in the management of Lyme disease, especially in areas where it is endemic or frequent. Avoiding tick-infested areas, wearing protective clothing (such as long sleeves and pants) when outdoors, using insect repellents containing DEET or permethrin, performing thorough tick checks after outdoor activities, and removing ticks as soon as possible with tweezers or a tick removal tool are all potential prevention strategies. Furthermore, landscaping activities such as establishing tick-safe zones and minimizing tick habitat near residences and recreational areas can help reduce the risk of tick exposure.

Conventional Lyme disease treatment options include a comprehensive strategy focused on eliminating the infection, treating symptoms, and boosting recovery. Antibiotic medication remains the foundation of treatment, augmented by symptomatic management, supportive treatments, follow-up care, and preventative initiatives. Individuals suffering from Lyme disease can achieve the best possible outcomes and continue a healthy, meaningful lifestyle with timely diagnosis, effective medication, and thorough care.

Working with Healthcare Providers on Lyme Disease Management

Navigating Lyme illness necessitates a joint effort between patients and healthcare professionals. From diagnosis to treatment and continuing maintenance, excellent communication and collaboration are critical to attaining the best results and improving overall well-being. In this thorough guide, we'll look at the most important parts of collaborating with healthcare professionals to treat Lyme disease, as well as practical ideas and insights for building a productive and helpful relationship.

1. Establishing Clear Communication

Open and open communication is essential for any effective patient-provider relationship. When dealing with Lyme disease, it is important to express your symptoms, concerns, and treatment choices openly and candidly. Be proactive in asking questions and getting answers regarding your diagnosis, treatment choices, and prognosis.

Additionally, offer input to your healthcare physician on how you're feeling and how your symptoms are developing. Maintaining good communication can ensure that you and your healthcare team are on the same page and working toward the same goals.

2. Seeking Experienced Providers

Finding healthcare experts who have expertise in identifying and treating Lyme disease is crucial. Look for practitioners who understand the complexity of Lyme disease, including its many symptoms and potential consequences. Consider consulting with experts such as infectious disease physicians, Lyme-literate doctors, or integrative medicine practitioners who understand tick-borne diseases and can provide complete therapy. Before committing to treatment, make sure to question potential physicians about their expertise and approach to Lyme disease care.

3. Advocating for Your Needs

As a patient, you must advocate for your own needs and preferences throughout the treatment process. Do not be reluctant to express your concerns, seek second views, or request different treatment alternatives if you believe they are essential. Remember that you are an active participant in your healthcare journey, and your feedback is valuable. Collaborate with your healthcare team to create a treatment plan that reflects your objectives, values, and lifestyle choices. By advocating for yourself, you can make sure your voice is heard and your healthcare requirements are met successfully.

4. Participating in Shared Decision-Making

Shared decision-making is a collaborative healthcare method in which patients and doctors work together to make informed treatment decisions. In the context of Lyme disease management, collaborative decision-making enables you to actively choose the optimal course of action for your treatment. Consider the advantages and disadvantages of various treatment alternatives, and balance them against your values and objectives. Discuss your preferences with your healthcare professional, and collaborate to create a plan that meets your unique requirements and preferences. Participating in shared decision-making might help you feel empowered and confident about your treatment options.

5. Staying Informed

Learning about Lyme disease and how to treat it is essential for making educated decisions and advocating for oneself. Stay current on the latest research, treatment guidelines, and developing medicines by consulting trustworthy sources such as medical journals, government health agencies, and patient advocacy groups. Be proactive in your search for information and tools that can help you better understand your illness and navigate the healthcare system successfully. Staying educated allows you to make informed decisions about your care and actively participate with your healthcare professionals in meaningful discussions about treatment options and methods.

6. Following Treatment Plans

Adherence to your treatment plan is critical for successful Lyme disease management. This may involve taking prescription medications as instructed, attending follow-up appointments, and adhering to the lifestyle advice made by your healthcare team. Maintain consistency with your treatment plan and express any obstacles or issues you experience along the way. Your healthcare practitioner can give assistance and direction to help you overcome barriers and stay on track with your treatment plan.

7. Addressing Mental Health Needs

Living with Lyme disease can hurt your mental and emotional health. Don't be afraid to seek treatment from mental health specialists who can guide you through the psychological issues that come with chronic disease. Discuss any anxiety, despair, or stress you are experiencing with your healthcare practitioner, as well as coping and resiliency skills. Remember that treating your mental health issues is an important element of comprehensive Lyme disease care and can lead to a higher quality of life.

8. Maintaining Engagement in Your Care

Staying actively involved in your healthcare journey is critical to effective Lyme disease treatment. Keep a record of your symptoms, treatment progress, and any changes in your condition. Maintain open contact with your healthcare team, and schedule regular check-ins to address your continuing care requirements. By being involved and proactive, you may actively manage your Lyme disease and move toward better health and well-being.

Finally, successful Lyme disease management requires collaboration with healthcare providers. You can improve your treatment outcomes and overall wellness by establishing clear communication, seeking experienced providers, advocating for your needs, participating in shared decision-making, staying informed, adhering to treatment plans, addressing mental health needs, and remaining engaged in your care. Remember that you are not alone in your journey, and your healthcare team will assist you every step of the way.

Accessing Support Services

Accessing support services is a crucial aspect of handling Lyme disease successfully. From medical care to emotional support, getting a range of services can help people deal with the challenges of living with this complex illness. Here's a closer look at some key support programs offered to those affected by Lyme disease:

1. Medical Care

Medical care forms the basis of Lyme disease treatment. Accessing healthcare services from experienced professionals, such as primary care doctors, infectious disease experts, and integrative medicine practitioners, is important for evaluation, treatment, and ongoing tracking of the condition.

Seeking medical care quickly can lead to early discovery and intervention, which is crucial for avoiding complications and boosting healing.

2. Lyme-Literate Healthcare Providers

Finding healthcare providers who are informed about Lyme disease, often referred to as Lyme-literate doctors can be helpful. These professionals have experience identifying and treating Lyme disease and other tick-borne illnesses, and they stay informed on the latest research and treatment recommendations. Working with a Lyme-literate healthcare provider can guarantee that people receive comprehensive and personalized care tailored to their unique needs.

3. Support Groups

Joining a support group for Lyme disease can provide useful mental support, practical help, and a sense of community for people living with the illness. Support groups offer a safe place for sharing experiences, asking questions, and connecting with others who understand the difficulties of Lyme disease directly. Whether in-person or online, support groups can offer useful tools and encouragement for those managing the complexities of Lyme disease.

4. Mental Health Services

Living with Lyme disease can take a toll on mental health, leading to feelings of stress, worry, sadness, and isolation. Accessing mental health services, such as counseling, therapy, or support from a psychologist or therapist, can help people deal with the emotional challenges of chronic sickness. Mental health experts can provide methods for managing stress, better coping skills, and enhancing general well-being.

5. Patient Advocacy Organizations

Patient advocacy organizations committed to Lyme disease provide a wealth of tools, information, and support for people affected by the condition. These groups often offer teaching tools, online platforms, helplines, and lobbying efforts to raise awareness and support research into Lyme disease.

Connecting with patient support organizations can empower people to become informed champions for themselves and others living with Lyme disease.

6. Alternative Therapies

Exploring alternative therapies and complementary techniques can support traditional medical care for Lyme disease. Techniques such as acupuncture, massage treatment, chiropractic care, and herbal medicine may offer disease relief, stress reduction, and general health support. It's important to speak with healthcare professionals before incorporating alternative therapies into your treatment plan to ensure safety and success.

7. Educational Resources

Accessing reliable educational tools about Lyme disease can enable people to become informed advocates for their health. Reputable websites, books, articles, and educational materials given by healthcare organizations and patient support groups can offer useful information about Lyme disease symptoms, diagnosis, treatment choices, prevention strategies, and coping techniques. Staying informed can help people make informed choices about their care and handle the challenges of living with Lyme disease.

In conclusion, getting support services is important for people living with Lyme disease to manage their condition effectively and improve their quality of life.

Whether through medical care, support groups, mental health services, patient advocacy organizations, alternative therapies, or educational resources, seeking out a range of support services can provide individuals with the tools, resources, and support they need to navigate the challenges of living with Lyme disease.

Chapter 6: Lifestyle Adjustments

Making lifestyle changes is important for people managing Lyme disease. This may involve changing daily routines, dietary habits, and physical activities to fit symptoms and promote general well-being. Incorporating rest methods, such as mindfulness meditation or gentle yoga, can help handle stress and support healing.

Prioritizing sleep hygiene and keeping a balanced diet rich in nutrients can also support immune function and improve energy levels. Additionally, avoiding possible causes, such as environmental toxins or certain foods, can reduce symptom worsening. By making careful lifestyle changes, individuals with Lyme disease can improve their quality of life and better control their condition.

Exercise and Movement in Lyme Disease Management

Exercise and movement play a vital role in general health and well-being, even for people living with chronic diseases such as Lyme disease. While it's important to approach exercise with care and adapt activities to individual capabilities and symptoms, incorporating regular movement into daily life can have numerous benefits for those managing Lyme disease.

In this comprehensive guide, we'll explore the value of exercise and movement, safe and effective methods for incorporating physical activity, and the possible impact on symptoms and general quality of life.

The Importance of Exercise

Regular exercise offers a variety of benefits for people with Lyme disease, including:

1. Improved Physical Health

Exercise strengthens muscles, improves cardiovascular health, and enhances flexibility and movement, which can help people better handle the physical challenges associated with Lyme disease.

2. Enhanced Mood and Mental Health

Physical exercise produces endorphins, neurotransmitters that promote feelings of happiness and well-being. Exercise also lowers stress, worry, and sadness, common symptoms experienced by people with chronic diseases like Lyme disease.

3. Better Sleep Quality

Engaging in regular physical exercise can improve sleep quality and length, which is important for general health and immune function. Adequate restorative sleep supports the body's mending processes and helps lower inflammation and pain linked with Lyme disease.

4. Increased Energy Levels

While fatigue is a typical sign of Lyme disease, light exercise can strangely improve energy levels by better circulation through oxygenation, and nutrient delivery to cells throughout the body.

5. Enhanced Immune Function Moderate

exercise has been shown to support immune function by boosting the circulation of immune cells and improving the body's ability to fight off infections and diseases, including Lyme disease.

Safe and Effective Exercise Strategies

When adding exercise to a Lyme disto management plan, it's important to value safety and listen to your body's signals. Here are some tips for safe and successful exercise:

1. Start Slowly

Begin with gentle, low-impact exercises such as walking, swimming, or tai chi, and gradually increase energy and time as allowed.

2. Listen to Your Body

Pay attention to how your body responds to exercise and change actions accordingly. If you experience greater pain, tiredness, or other symptoms, scale back or change your workout routine.

3. Focus on Flexibility and Strength

Incorporate stretching routines and strength training to improve flexibility, joint stability, and muscle tone. Resistance bands, bodyweight exercises, and yoga can be useful choices.

4. Choose Low-Impact Activities

Opt for activities that are easy on the joints and muscles, such as riding, water yoga, or using elliptical machines. Avoid high-impact tasks that may worsen joint pain or inflammation.

5. Prioritize Rest and Recovery

Allow time for rest and recovery between exercise sessions to avoid overexertion and reduce the risk of injury. Listen to your body's cues and plan rest days as needed.

6. Stay Fresh

Drink plenty of water before, during, and after exercise to stay fresh and support the best performance. Dehydration can worsen fatigue and other symptoms linked with Lyme disease.

7. Seek Professional Guidance

Consult with a healthcare provider or physical trainer skilled in working with people with chronic illnesses to build a safe and personalized exercise plan. They can provide advice on suitable activities, modifications, and precautions based on your particular needs and limits.

Impact on Symptoms and Quality of Life

Regular exercise has been shown to have a good effect on symptoms and general quality of life for individuals living with Lyme disease:

1. Pain Management

Exercise can help lower pain by promoting the

release of endorphins, improving circulation, and increasing muscle strength and flexibility. It can also distract from pain feelings and improve mood, making it easier to deal with discomfort.

2. Fatigue Reduction

While it may seem counterintuitive, gentle exercise can help tiredness by increasing energy levels and improving general stamina. Engaging in regular physical exercise can also promote better sleep quality, which is important for fighting tiredness and recovering energy levels.

3. Mood Enhancement

Physical exercise has been shown to have antidepressant and anxiolytic effects, making it an effective tool for controlling mood disorders such as sadness and anxiety. Exercise produces neurotransmitters like serotonin and dopamine, which are linked with feelings of happiness and relaxation.

4. Functional Improvement

By improving strength, flexibility, and cardiovascular fitness, exercise can improve functional skills and make everyday tasks and activities of daily living (ADLs) easier to perform. This can lead to greater freedom and a better quality of life for people with Lyme disease.

Incorporating Movement into Daily Life

In addition to structured exercise sessions, it's important to bring movement into everyday life to support general health and well-being:

1. Stay Active Throughout the Day
Look for chances to move and stretch throughout the day, such as taking short walks, standing up and stretching regularly, or doing household jobs.

2. Make Movement Enjoyable
Find things that you enjoy and that fit your hobbies and preferences. Whether it's dancing, farming, or

playing with pets, make moving a fun and enjoyable part of your daily routine.

3. Set Realistic Goals

Set realistic and doable goals for physical exercise, taking into account your present fitness level, symptoms, and limits. Celebrate small wins and growth along the way.

4. Listen to Your Body

Be aware of your body's cues and change your exercise level and intensity accordingly. Honor your boundaries and value self-care when needed.

Exercise and movement play a key role in controlling Lyme disease and supporting general health and well-being. By incorporating safe and effective exercise methods into daily life, people with Lyme disease can experience changes in physical health, mood, sleep quality, and general quality of life.

Prioritizing regular physical activity, listening to your body's signals, and getting professional advice when needed can help people with Lyme disease reap the numerous benefits of exercise while minimizing the risk of exacerbating symptoms or causing harm. Remember that every step counts, and even small amounts o movement can make a significant difference in controlling Lyme disease and living life to the best.

Sleep Hygiene in Lyme Disease Management

Quality sleep is important for general health and well-being, especially for people managing Lyme disease. Sleep hygiene refers to the habits and practices that promote good sleep patterns and improve the quality and length of sleep. In this thorough guide, we'll explore the importance of sleep hygiene in Lyme disease treatment, common sleep problems associated with the condition, and practical tips for improving sleep quality and amount.

The Importance of Sleep in Lyme Disease Management

Quality sleep is important for people with Lyme disease for several reasons:

1. Supports Healing

Adequate and restorative sleep supports the body's healing processes, including immune function, tissue repair, and hormone control. Quality sleep is important for fighting inflammation and boosting healing from Lyme disease.

2. Improves Symptom Management

Sleep plays a key role in controlling symptoms linked with Lyme disease, such as pain, fatigue, and cognitive impairment. Quality sleep can lower symptom intensity and improve the general quality of life for people dealing with the condition.

3. Enhances Mental Health

Sleep is closely linked to mental health, and poor sleep can worsen symptoms of anxiety, sadness, and mood disorders widely experienced by people with chronic illnesses like Lyme disease.

Prioritizing sound sleep can support mental well-being and resilience.

4. Optimizes Energy Levels

Restorative sleep helps restore energy stores and fight tiredness, a common sign of Lyme disease. Quality sleep can improve everyday alertness, focus, and cognitive function, allowing people to better handle daily tasks and responsibilities.

Common Sleep Disturbances in Lyme Disease

Individuals with Lyme disease may experience different sleep problems, including:

1. Insomnia

Difficulty getting asleep, staying asleep, or waking up too early is common among people with Lyme disease. Insomnia can be caused by pain, discomfort, worry, or drug side effects.

2. Restless Leg Syndrome (RLS)

RLS is defined by uncomfortable feelings in the legs and an irresistible urge to move them, often leading to disturbed sleep. RLS may be worsened by Lyme disease-related inflammation or nerve damage.

3. Sleep Disordered Breathing

Sleep apnea and other kinds of sleep-disordered breathing can occur in people with Lyme disease, leading to pauses in breathing during sleep and daytime tiredness. Sleep-disordered breathing may be linked to inflammation, muscle weakness, or central nervous system failure.

4. Fragmented Sleep

Individuals with Lyme disease may experience disrupted sleep patterns marked by frequent awakenings throughout the night. Fragmented sleep can result from pain, fatigue, nocturia (frequent urination), or drug effects.

Practical Tips for Improving Sleep Hygiene

Improving sleep hygiene can help people with Lyme disease improve their sleep quality and length. Here are some useful tips:

1. Establish a Consistent Sleep Schedule

Go to bed and wake up at the same time each day, even on weekends, to regulate your body's internal clock and support a normal sleep-wake cycle.

2. Create a Relaxing Bedtime Routine

Develop a relaxing pre-sleep practice to signal to your body that it's time to wind down. Activities such as reading, listening to calming music, or practicing relaxation methods like deep breathing or meditation can help prepare your mind and body for sleep.

3. Create a Comfortable Sleep Environment

Make your bedroom suitable for sleep by keeping it cool, dark, and quiet. Invest in a comfortable mattress and pillows, and consider using white noise makers or earplugs to block out annoying noise.

4. Limit Stimulants and Electronics

Avoid coffee, smoking, and stimulating activities (e.g., exercise, screen time) close to bedtime, as they can interfere with sleep start and quality. Minimize exposure to screens (e.g., smartphones, computers) before bed, as the blue light released can upset circadian rhythms and melatonin production.

5. Manage Pain and Discomfort

Address any pain or discomfort that may disrupt sleep by using supportive pillows or mattress toppers, practicing relaxation techniques, or taking pain-relieving medicines as recommended.

6. Address Anxiety and Stress

Manage worry and stress with breathing techniques, cognitive-behavioral therapy, or mindfulness routines. Consider keeping a stress book to jot down any racing thoughts before bed, allowing your mind to relax and let go of concerns.

7. Limit Daytime Naps

While short, restful naps can be helpful, avoid long or late afternoon naps that may interfere with nighttime sleep. If you feel the need to nap, try for a short nap (20-30 minutes) earlier in the day to avoid disrupting your sleep-wake routine.

8. Seek Professional Help if Needed

If sleep disturbances continue despite adopting sleep hygiene strategies, speak with a healthcare provider or sleep specialist. They can examine underlying reasons for sleep disturbances and suggest suitable treatments, such as medication adjustments or cognitive-behavioral therapy for insomnia (CBT-I).

Quality sleep is important for people with Lyme disease to support healing, symptom management, and general well-being. By prioritizing sleep hygiene and adopting realistic methods to improve sleep quality and duration, people with Lyme disease can enhance their sleep habits and enjoy the numerous benefits of restorative sleep. Remember that consistency and patience are key when it comes to better sleep hygiene, and small changes can lead to major gains in sleep quality and general quality of life.

Stress Management Techniques for Treatment of Lyme Disease

Living with Lyme disease may be difficult, and managing stress is essential for general health and symptom management. Individuals with Lyme disease might benefit from stress management approaches to help them deal with the physical, emotional, and psychological obstacles that come with the condition. In this thorough book, we'll look at numerous stress management approaches and practical tactics for incorporating them into everyday life to encourage resilience, relaxation, and a higher quality of life.

Importance of Stress Management

Chronic stress can aggravate symptoms and have an influence on overall health in Lyme disease patients. Stress causes the production of chemicals like cortisol and adrenaline, which can exacerbate inflammation, weaken the immune system, and contribute to symptoms like pain, exhaustion, and cognitive impairment. Individuals with Lyme disease can lessen the negative impacts of stress on their health and well-being by practicing stress management practices, as well as enhancing their capacity to cope with the condition's challenges.

Stress Management Techniques

1. Mindfulness Meditation

Mindfulness meditation entails focusing on the present moment without judgment, allowing people to notice their thoughts, feelings, and sensations without becoming overwhelmed by them. Regular mindfulness practice can help decrease stress, increase relaxation, and improve general well-being. Simple mindfulness techniques, inc including breathing, body scans, and guided meditation, can be used regularly for awareness and resilience.

2. Deep Breathing Exercises

Deep breathing exercises, sometimes called diaphragmatic or abdominal breathing, include taking slow, deep breaths to trigger the body's relaxation response. Deep breathing helps alleviate tension, decrease blood pressure, and induce relaxation. Deep breathing exercises should be practiced throughout the day, especially during times of high stress or worry, to quiet the nervous system and generate a state of serenity.

3. Progressive Muscular Relaxation (PMR)

Progressive muscle relaxation is a method that includes tensing and then releasing various muscle groups throughout the body to induce physical relaxation and stress relief. Individuals can alleviate physical tension and achieve a deep sensation of relaxation by gradually releasing muscle groups from head to toe. Practice PMR on a daidailyally before bedtime, to improve peaceful sleep and minimize muscular tension caused by stress.

4. Yoga and Stretch

Yoga combines physical postures, breathing methods, and mindfulness practices to help you relax, be more flexible, and relieve stress. Gentle yoga and stretching activities can help relieve muscular tension, improve circulation, and boost general health. Incorporate yoga into your everyday practice, emphasizing moderate, restorative positions that promote relaxation and stress reduction.

5. Exercise and Physical Activity

Regular exercise is a great method to decrease stress, enhance mood, and promote overall health and wellness. Engage in enjoyable activities such as walking, cycling, swimming, or dancing to increase endorphin levels and reduce stress. Aim for at least 30 minutes of moderate-intensity exercise every day of the week to gain the advantages of physical activity for stress management and symptom reduction.

6. Creative Expression

Taking part in creative hobbies like painting, writing, music, or gardening can help you express yourself and relieve stress. Creative expression enables people to channel their emotions and experiences into meaningful and pleasant activities that promote relaxation and well-being. Find creative activities that appeal to you and incorporate them into your daily routine to decrease stress and improve mood.

7. Social Support

Connecting with helpful friends, family members, or peers can help you cope with stress both emotionally and practically. Share your experiences, worries, and emotions with trusted people who can provide empathy, support, and understanding. Join Lyme disease support groups or online forums to connect with people who have faced similar struggles and experiences.

8. Healthy Lifestyle Habits

Prioritize healthy lifestyle practices including eating a well-balanced diet, getting enough sleep, staying hydrated, and avoiding excessive alcohol and caffeine use. These routines promote general health and resilience, making it simpler to cope with stress and manage Lyme disease symptoms.

Stress management strategies are important in Lyme disease management because they help people deal with the physical, emotional, and psychological obstacles that come with the condition. Individuals with Lyme disease can lessen the harmful impacts of stress on their health and well-being by implementing stress management practices into their everyday lives, improving their capacity to cope with the condition's problems.

Remember that stress management is a skill that takes time and practice, and even minor modifications may lead to big increases in overall resilience and quality of life. Individuals with Lyme disease who include stress management practices in their everyday lives see stress on their health and well-being while also improving their capacity to cope with the condition's challenges.

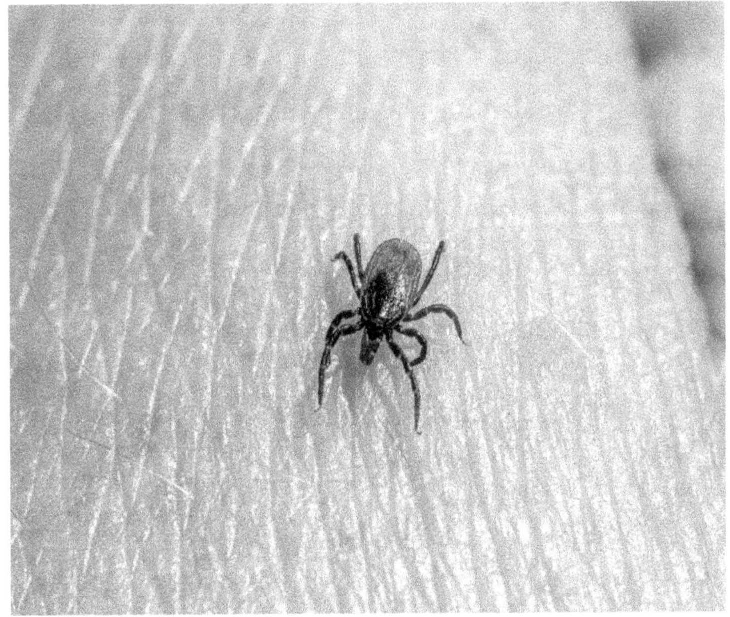

Conclusion

Finally, Lyme disease comets its own set of problems that can affect all parts of daily life, from your physical health to your mental health. In this complete guide, we've talked about many aspects of managing Lyme disease, such as its signs, diagnosis, treatment choices, lifestyle changes, and ways to deal with stress. We can help people with Lyme disease get through the difficult parts of life and improve their general quality of life by giving them information, useful tips, and support.

A complicated illness called Lyme disease, also known as the "great imitator," is spread by the bite of an infected tick. The bacterial agent responsible for this illness is Borrelia burgdorferi. The disease can show up in many different ways, such as tiredness, joint pain, memory loss, and problems with the nervous system. Early diagnosis and treatment are very important for avoiding long-term problems and speeding up the healing process.

Lyme disease is usually treated in several ways, such as with several kills the underlying infections, supportive treatments to ease symptoms, and changes to a person's lifestyle to improve their general health. Additionally, complementary and alternative treatments, such as herbal medicines, acupuncture, and dietary changes, may offer additional support and symptom relief for people with Lyme disease.

Making lifestyle changes is important for people managing Lyme disease. This may involve changing daily routines, dietary habits, and physical activities to fit symptoms and promote general well-being. Prioritizing rest, relaxation, and self-care can help people deal with the challenges of living with Lyme disease and keep a sense of balance and resilience.

Stress management techniques are vital for people with Lyme disease to deal with the physical, emotional, and psychological challenges involved with the condition. Mindfulness meditation, deep breathing techniques, gradual muscle relaxation, and yoga can promote relaxation, reduce stress, and improve general well-being. Engaging in artistic expression, finding social support, and prioritizing healthy living habits are also effective tactics for managing stress and boosting resiliency.

As we look ahead, it's important to continue raising knowledge about Lyme disease, advocating for better diagnostics and treatment choices, and supporting people affected by the condition. By creating a better understanding of Lyme disease within the medical community and society at large, we can reduce stigma, increase access to care, and improve outcomes for those living with the illness.

Ultimately, our goal is to enable people with Lyme disease to take an active role in their health and well-being. By giving access to comprehensive information, tools, and support services, we can help people make informed choices about their care, fight for their needs, and navigate the complexities of living with Lyme disease with confidence and resilience.

In closing, managing life with Lyme disease takes patience, resilience, and a caring group. By coming together to share information, experiences, and tools, we can create a more compassionate and understanding atmosphere for people living with Lyme disease. Together, we can help one another on the path to better health and well-being, ensuring that no one faces the challenges of Lyme disease alone.

As we end this guide, let us remember that each individual's journey with Lyme disease is unique, and there is no one-size-fits-all method for management. By accepting diversity understanding, and teamwork, we can create a more open and helpful community for people impacted by Lyme disease and foster hope for a better future.

Thank you for joining us on this journey, and may we continue to work together toward a world where everyone toward disease gets the care, support, and understanding they deserve.

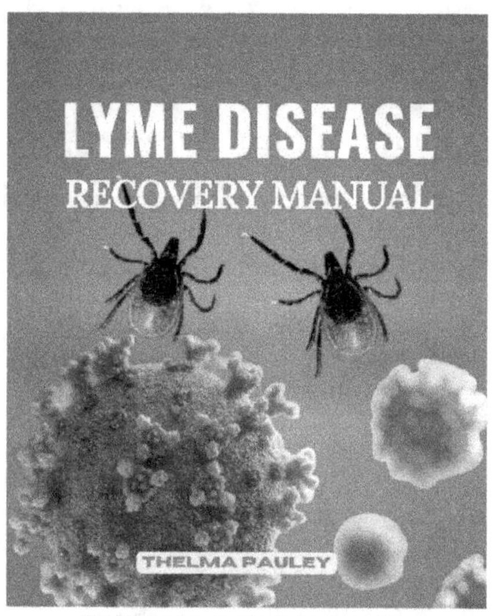

www.ingramcontent.com/pod-product-compliance
Lightning Source LLC
Chambersburg PA
CBHW070812260726
48660CB00005B/1828